Life Changer Interactive Journal

Kimberly Bozeman

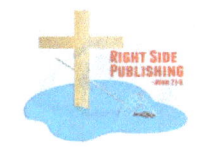

Right side publishing

Copyright 2020 by Kimberly Bozeman

All rights reserved. No part of this publication may be reproduced, distributed, or transmitted in any form or by any means, including photocopying, recording, or other electronic or mechanical methods, without the prior written permission of the publisher, except in the case of brief quotations embodied in critical reviews and certain other noncommercial uses permitted by copyright law. For permission requests, Email author addressed "Attention: Permissions,

Please contact Author Kimberly Bozeman for speaking engagements and all other permission request at healthyemotes@yahoo.com

ISBN 978-0-998864440
Library of Congress Control Number: 2020919203
Cover design by Tiny Rhodes /Tiny communications LLC

Edited by Elizabeth Morris

Layout by Felicia S. Cauley/Robert A. Cauley

Right Side Publishing
P.0 Box 339
Reynoldsburg, OH 43068
www.rightsidepublishing.com

ACKNOWLEDGEMENTS

I acknowledge my call and duty to serve as well as to help people on their journey called life. It is a wonderful honor and privilege to be instrumental in assisting individuals become a better version of themselves, walking in wholeness and victory!

I am thankful for my husband, Bishop Marvin C. Bozeman, for his encouragement and support. Thank you to my beloved mother for her relentless prayers and encouragement! I am grateful for my beautiful children; Larry, Camille, and William, also my grandchildren. I want to thank Bishop Fred Marshall for believing in me and for providing a wonderful opportunity to serve others. I would also like to acknowledge MarVon Forte who selflessly provides her artistic abilities, ideas, and time. Thank you to Robert and Brittany Bozeman for your supporting love. Also, appreciation to Koraya Scott for your artistic abilities and designs.

Most importantly, I acknowledge and dedicate this journal to the memory of my father, LeRoy Victor Trout, who always encouraged me to remain patient and consistent in reaching my goals. Finally, I acknowledge my siblings Angela, Vickie, and Tony. To God be the glory!

Contents

Acknowledgements iii
Introduction 1
How To Use This Journal 3
I Am Becoming Who I Shall Become! 4
Transformation Awaits You As The Sun Waits On The Dawning Of A New Day! 7
Create A Wonderful Day! 10
If It's Important Enough To Bother You, It's Important Enough To Discuss! 13
You Have The Ability To Create Your Own Atmosphere And Mood! 16
You Can't Grow In The Status Quo! 19
If You Change Your Mind, You Can Change Your Life! 22
Live While You're Living! 25
Whatever You Don't Address, You Give Permission To Exist! 28
Where There's Fruit, There Are Roots! 31
If You Don't Deal With Your Past, Your Past Will Deal With You! 34
What You Focus On, You Empower! 37
A House Divided Cannot Stand! Who You Need Is You! 40
Forgiveness Is The Key To Unlocking The Ball And Chain! 43
Compare Yourself To Yourself For Measureable Growth! 46
Creating A Better Version Of Self Derives From Within! 49
Love Yourself Unconditionally. Embrace Your Hidden Self! 52
Stop Perpetuating The Abandonment Cycle. Be There For You Now! 55
Do Not Say Things To Yourself That You Would Not Want Other People To Say To You! 58
Everyone Has Some Good Qualities. What Are Some Of Yours? 61
You Have Paid The "Guilt" Sentence For Too Long! Today Is Your Day Of Parole! Live Free! 64
Today Is Your Day Of A Turnaround! 67
Just As Currency Is Not Reduced Because It Has Been Lost, Tossed, Stepped On, Stepped Over, And Torn; Your Value Is Not Reduced Throughout Your Lifespan Due To Life's Circumstances! Know Your Worth! 70
This Circumstance Is Only A Moment In Time. It Is Not My Eternity! 73
When Emotions Are High, Slow Down And Breathe. You Will Be Able To Think A Little Clearer, And Your Consequences Will Be A Little Lighter. 76
Change Is Hard But Doable! 79
Just Because You Think A Thought, Does Not Mean The Thought Is Right! 82
Awareness Illuminates Your Path 85
Whatever You Do, Do It Wholeheartedly With Passion. Be The Experience! 88

Accept It. Sit With It. Keep It Moving! Ask! 91
Rain Is Your Opportunity To Grow, Be Nurtured, And Bloom! 94
You Can Have A Diagnosis, As Long As The Diagnosis Does Not Have You! 97
Do Not Dwell In The Camp Of Negativity! 100
Press Past Your Pain! 103
Forgiveness Benefits Me! 106
Validate Your Emotions. Don't Wait On Others To Validate Them For You! 109
Secret Pain Perpetuates A Destructive Cycle. Use Your Voice! 112
The Journey Towards Your Greater Self Entails Both Hills And Valleys. 115
Being Free Requires Forgiveness Of Self And Others. Choose Freedom! 118
Thoughts = Feelings Feelings = Behaviors Behaviors = Consequences 121
Is Your Desire To Change Greater Than Your Desire To Remain The Same? 124
You Are The Master Architect Of Your Life! Are You Constructive Or Destructive? 127
Emotional Healing Requires Vulnerability. 130
As Long As You Are Inhaling And Exhaling, You Can Begin Again. 133
What Others Think About You Is Not As Important As What You Think About Yourself! 136
It's Ok To Have Anger When Anger Does Not Have You! 139
Vvr! Value, Validate, And Respect Yourself! 142
Wholeness Begins Within! 145
Take Time Today To Breathe Deeply! 148
Exercise: Inhale Through The Nose For A Count Of Four. Hold For A Count Of Seven. 148
Exhale Slowly For A Count Of Eight. Four Rounds At A Time. 148
What Are You Grateful For? 151
Ground Yourself With Mindfulness! 154
The Voice Of Your Inner Critic Has A Big Mouth! Silence Its Voice With Love! 158
One Of The Greatest Relationships You Can Have Is The Relationship With Yourself! 161
Food Is Mood And Medicine 164
What Are You Eating? 164
To Move Forward, Radically Accept Your Current Circumstance! 167
Allow Pain To Push You Into Your Purpose! 170
As Plants Need Dirt To Grow, So Do We. Do Not Despise Your Dirty Places! 173
Plant Seeds Of Faith, And Hope In Your Subconscious Garden 176
Following Your Negative Emotions Will Take You Down A Destructive Path! 179
Pain Is The Master Teacher! What Lessons Have You Learned? 182
Love I Am Worthy Of Love, I Am Loving And Lovable! I Am Strong Enough To Give Love, ... 185
I Am Gracious To Receive Love! Love 185
Positive Distractions List 188
My Feelings List 190

INTRODUCTION

This is an interactive and transformative journal. This journal allows someone to recognize, identify, and process feelings and behaviors. One of my mottos is as follows: "Whatever you don't address, you give permission to exist!" Just because you suppress or ignore a problem does not mean that it goes away. As a matter of fact, you push it down inside of you, and it then becomes a part of you. Then, it takes up residence in every cell of your being. This is why some people may experience recurrent dreams, nightmares, and intrusive thoughts! Take my word for it; if you don't deal with it, IT will deal with you!

This journal helps you get frustration and pain out of your heart and head, and to put it onto paper! It is better out than in. One of the problems with human beings is that we do not like to be uncomfortable. I am asking you to become comfortable with getting uncomfortable! It is the healthiest way to heal.

Let me introduce the acronym *A.S.K. A* is for radical *A*cceptance. Life happens to all of us at one time or another. Things will come our way that we do not want to experience. Instead, we attempt to analyze and figure out why and how it happened. This increases stress and depression. You send messages to your sympathetic nervous system, and your adrenal glands release adrenaline and cortisol causing you to feel anxious, fearful and depressed. What we must realize is that there is absolutely nothing we can do about something that has already happened! No matter how much worrying, crying, and regretting you do; it has already happened. Accept it and decide to move forward. In other words, this is your new normal, hence radical *A*cceptance.

S is for *S*itting with it! It is absolutely okay to sit with the pain long enough to be more accepting of the current conditions. Sitting with it to have non-judgmental thoughts and allowing what is to just be. Sitting with the anger, disappointment, frustration, etc. to be open, honest, and validate your needs. When we sit with the uncomfortable experience, we are not suppressing but processing in a healthy way. For example, if you were adopted, you may have questions regarding the decisions of your biological parents. Understandably, these questions can be difficult and uncomfortable. However, this journal will help you to identify and sit with the emotions of abandonment, unworthiness, betrayal, etc. It will help you to cultivate and nurture your inner child. What you must realize at this time in your life, who you need now is **you**! You do not want to perpetuate the abandonment or abusive cycle. You must be at home for you now! You have the power to heal yourself, but you must first sit with yourself!

K, is for *K*eep it moving! You have heard the saying, "Analysis is paralysis!". You have to keep it moving, but how you proceed is very important! Will you proceed weighed down with extra weight, or will you be free? This question is a matter of choice and work! If you choose to be free, that means you must put in the work. Whereas if you choose the former, just do nothing! This journal will help you to get rid of the extra baggage or weight that impedes your emotional freedom and growth. By helping

Life Changer Interactive Journal

you to sort out your thoughts, feelings, and behaviors; this journal will provide better consequences and immeasurable growth!

Dare to be different, dare to grow, and dare to become a better version of yourself. Compare yourself only to yourself. Remember, you are in the process of becoming who you shall become!

HOW TO USE THIS JOURNAL

Openness and honesty are both effective and efficient. Remember the purpose of this journal is to help you change your mood and atmosphere. Identifying your thoughts and triggers are a paramount part of the process towards change. You may visit the back of the book to assist you in properly identifying and labeling your feelings. Go to the "Feelings List" to choose what feeling relates closest to what you are experiencing and fill in the blanks. You also have a "Positive Distractions" list to assist you in reducing stress, worry, anxiety, fear, etc. These positive distractions will also help you to feel better, since thoughts send signals to your brain to release corresponding chemical reactions. Good thoughts equate good feelings, just as bad thoughts lead to bad feelings. Choose from the positive distractions list or be creative and make up your own but ENJOY THE PROCESS!

I AM BECOMING WHO I SHALL BECOME!

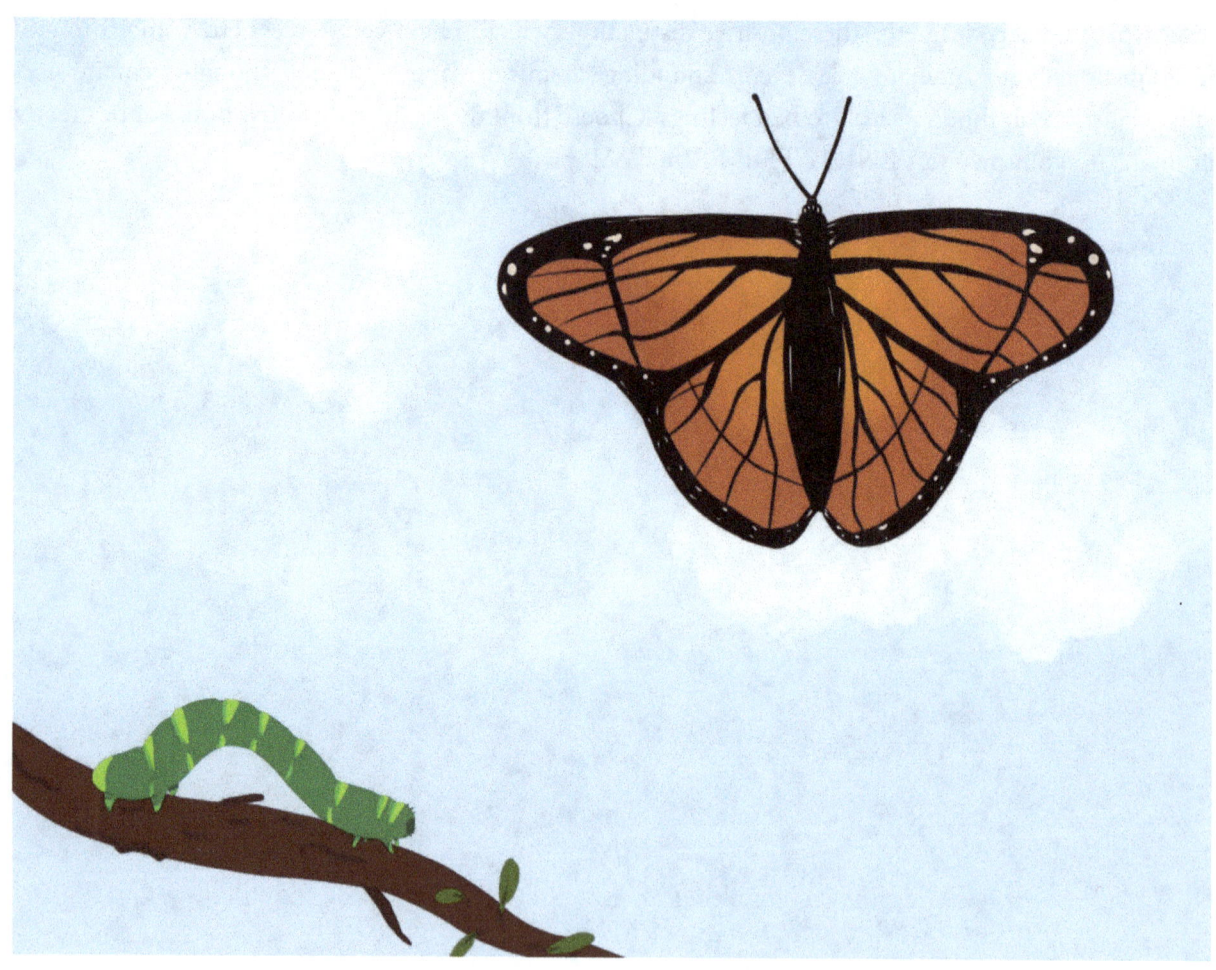

#1 DATE:

Right now, I feel _____. I know/do not know (circle one) what triggered this feeling. My triggers as I know them are

_____

_____

_____

_____

WHERE ARE MY THOUGHTS?

My thoughts are focused on my past/present/future (circle one), and they consist

_____

_____

_____

_____

To Feel Better I Will:

a) Choose the opposite behavior. (Use positive distractions list.)

b) Challenge my thoughts. (Just because I think a thought does not mean it's right!)

c) Limit access to triggers.

d) Silence my inner critic with positive self-talk.

e) Use coping skills. _____

_____

What Are My New Actions?

    a) New beliefs and thoughts about the situation:

___

___

___

___

    b) My positive affirmations for today are:

___

___

___

TRANSFORMATION AWAITS YOU
AS THE SUN WAITS ON THE DAWNING
OF A NEW DAY!

#2 Date:

Right now, I feel _____. I know/do not know (circle one) what triggered this feeling. My triggers as I know them are_____.

_____

_____

_____

_____

WHERE ARE MY THOUGHTS?

My thoughts are focused on my past/present/future (circle one), and they consist of_____.

_____

_____

_____

_____

To Feel Better I Will:

a) Choose the opposite behavior. (Use positive distractions list.)

b) Challenge my thoughts. (Just because I think a thought does not mean it's right!)

c) Limit access to triggers.

d) Silence my inner critic with positive self-talk.

e) Use coping skills. _____

_____

What Are My New Actions?

    a) New beliefs and thoughts about the situation:

_____

_____

_____

_____

    b) My positive affirmations for today are:.

_____

_____

_____

_____

CREATE A WONDERFUL DAY!

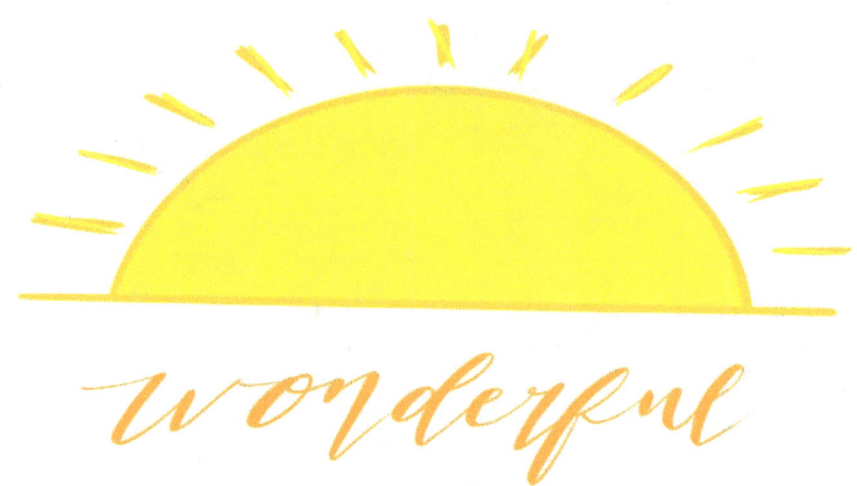

#3 Date:

Right now, I feel _____. I know/do not know (circle one) what triggered this feeling. My triggers as I know them are_____.

_____

_____

_____

WHERE ARE MY THOUGHTS?

My thoughts are focused on my past/present/future (circle one), and they consist of_____.

_____

_____

_____

To Feel Better I Will:

a) Choose the opposite behavior. (Use positive distractions list.)

b) Challenge my thoughts. (Just because I think a thought does not mean it's right!)

c) Limit access to triggers.

d) Silence my inner critic with positive self-talk.

e) Use coping skills. _____

Life Changer Interactive Journal

What Are My New Actions?

    a)   New beliefs and thoughts about the situation

_____

_____

_____

_____

    b)   My positive affirmations for today are:.

_____

_____

_____

_____

IF IT'S IMPORTANT ENOUGH TO BOTHER YOU, IT'S IMPORTANT ENOUGH TO DISCUSS!

#4 Date:

Right now, I feel _____. I know/do not know (circle one) what triggered this feeling. My triggers as I know them are_____.

_____

_____

_____

WHERE ARE MY THOUGHTS?

My thoughts are focused on my past/present/future (circle one), and they consist of_____.

_____

_____

_____

To Feel Better I Will:

a) Choose the opposite behavior. (Use positive distractions list.)

b) Challenge my thoughts. (Just because I think a thought does not mean it's right!)

c) Limit access to triggers.

d) Silence my inner critic with positive self-talk.

e) Use coping skills. _____

_____

What Are My New Actions?

    a) New beliefs and thoughts about the situation:

___

___

___

___

    b) My positive affirmations for today are:

___

___

___

You Have the Ability to Create Your Own Atmosphere and Mood!

1. Invite the sun into your environment.
2. Meditate.
3. Sing.
4. Listen to positive music.
5. Practice mindfulness.
6. Eat healthy foods.
7. Light candles.

#5 Date:

Right now, I feel _____. I know/do not know (circle one) what triggered this feeling. My triggers as I know them are_____.

_____

_____

_____

WHERE ARE MY THOUGHTS?

My thoughts are focused on my past/present/future (circle one), and they consist of_____.

_____

_____

_____

To Feel Better I Will:

    a) Choose the opposite behavior. (Use positive distractions list.)

    b) Challenge my thoughts. (Just because I think a thought does not mean it's right!)

    c) Limit access to triggers.

    d) Silence my inner critic with positive self-talk.

    e) Use coping skills. _____

Life Changer Interactive Journal

What Are My New Actions?

    a) New beliefs and thoughts about the situation:

    b) My positive affirmations for today are:

You Can't Grow in the Status Quo!

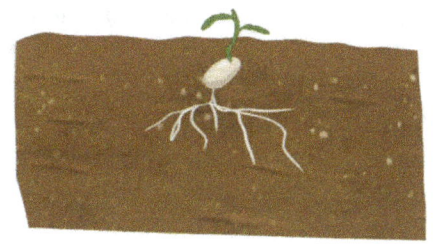

#6 Date:

Right now, I feel _____. I know/do not know (circle one) what triggered this feeling. My triggers as I know them are_____.

_____

_____

_____

WHERE ARE MY THOUGHTS?

My thoughts are focused on my past/present/future (circle one), and they consist of_____.

_____

_____

_____

To Feel Better, I Will:

    a) Choose the opposite behavior. (Use positive distractions list.)

    b) Challenge my thoughts. (Just because I think a thought does not mean it's right!)

    c) Limit access to triggers.

    d) Silence my inner critic with positive self-talk.

    e) Use coping skills. _____

What Are My New Actions?

    a) New beliefs and thoughts about the situation:

_____

_____

_____

_____

    b) My positive affirmations for today are:

_____

_____

_____

_____

IF YOU CHANGE YOUR MIND, YOU CAN CHANGE YOUR LIFE!

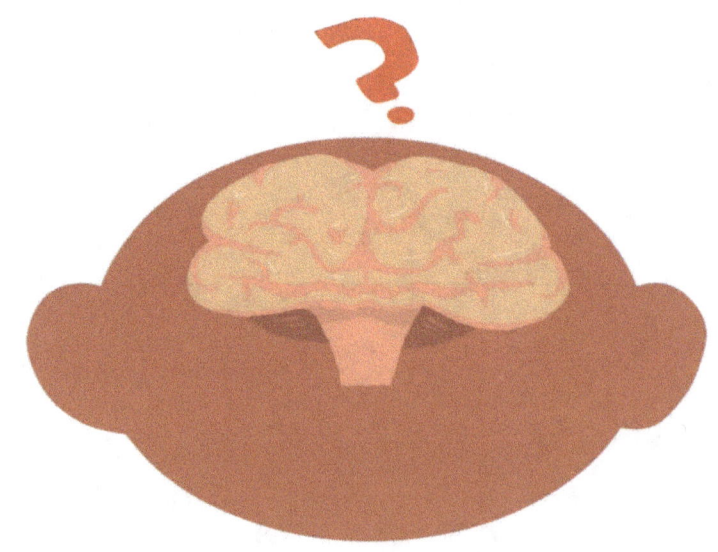

#7 Date:

Right now, I feel _____. I know/do not know (circle one) what triggered this feeling. My triggers as I know them are_____.

_____

_____

_____

WHERE ARE MY THOUGHTS?

My thoughts are focused on my past/present/future (circle one), and they consist of_____.

_____

_____

_____

To Feel Better I Will:

    a) Choose the opposite behavior. (Use positive distractions list.)

    b) Challenge my thought. (Just because I think a thought does not mean it's right!)

    c) Limit access to triggers.

    d) Silence my inner critic with positive self-talk.

    e) Use coping skills. _____

_____

What Are My New Actions?

    a)   New beliefs and thoughts about the situation:

___

___

___

___

    b)   My positive affirmations for today are:

___

___

___

___

LIVE WHILE YOU'RE LIVING!

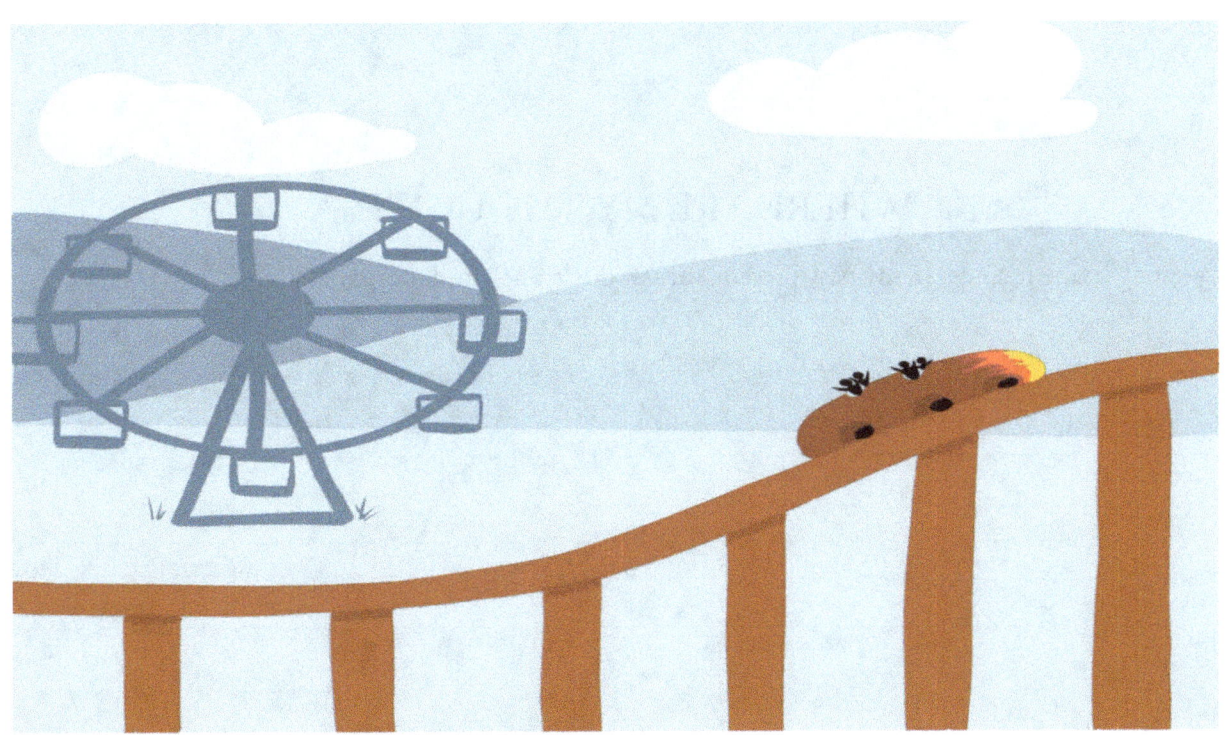

#8 Date:

Right now, I feel _____. I know/do not know (circle one) what triggered this feeling. My triggers as I know them are_____.

_____

_____

_____

WHERE ARE MY THOUGHTS?

My thoughts are focused on my past/present/future (circle one), and they consist of_____.

_____

_____

_____

To Feel Better I Will:

    a) Choose the opposite behavior. (Use positive distractions list.)

    b) Challenge my thoughts. (Just because I think a thought does not mean it's right!)

    c) Limit access to triggers.

    d) Silence my inner critic with positive self-talk.

    e) Use coping skill. _____

_____

What Are My New Actions?

    a)   New beliefs and thoughts about the situation:

___

___

___

___

    b)   My positive affirmations for today are:

___

___

___

___

WHATEVER YOU DON'T ADDRESS, YOU GIVE PERMISSION TO EXIST!

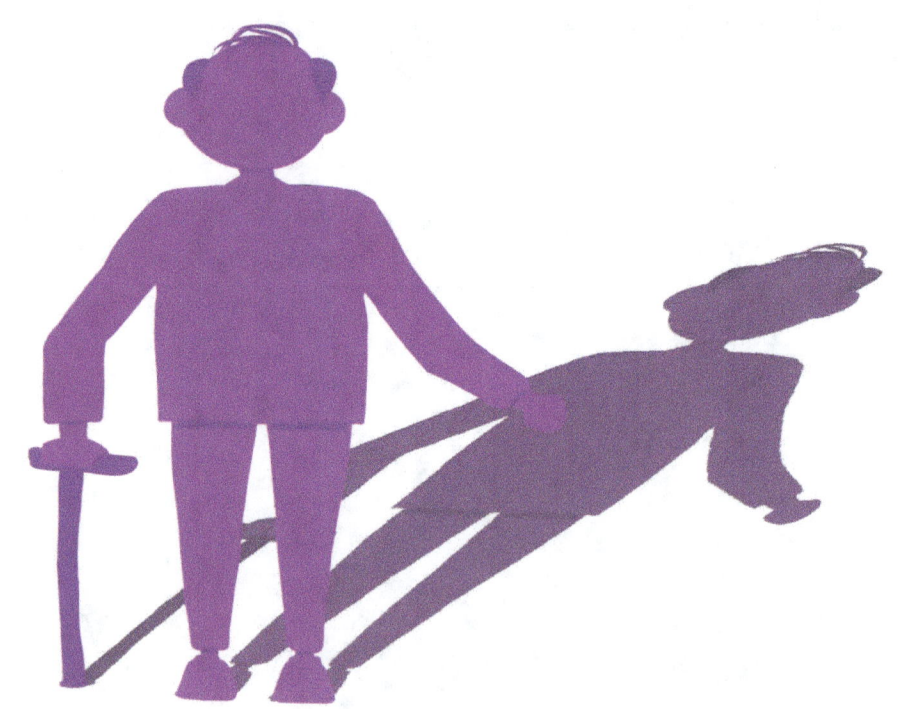

#9 Date:

Right now, I feel _____. I know/do not know (circle one) what triggered this feeling. My triggers as I know them are_____.

_____

_____

_____

_____

WHERE ARE MY THOUGHTS?

My thoughts are focused on my past/present/future (circle one), and they consist of_____.

_____

_____

_____

_____

To Feel Better I Will:

a) Choose the opposite behavior. (Use positive distractions list.)

b) Challenge my thoughts. (Just because I think a thought does not mean it's right!)

c) Limit access to triggers.

d) Silence my inner critic with positive self-talk.

e) Use coping skills. _____

_____

What Are My New Actions?

a) New beliefs and thoughts about the situation:

___

___

___

___

b) My positive affirmations for today are:

___

___

___

___

Where There's Fruit, There Are Roots!

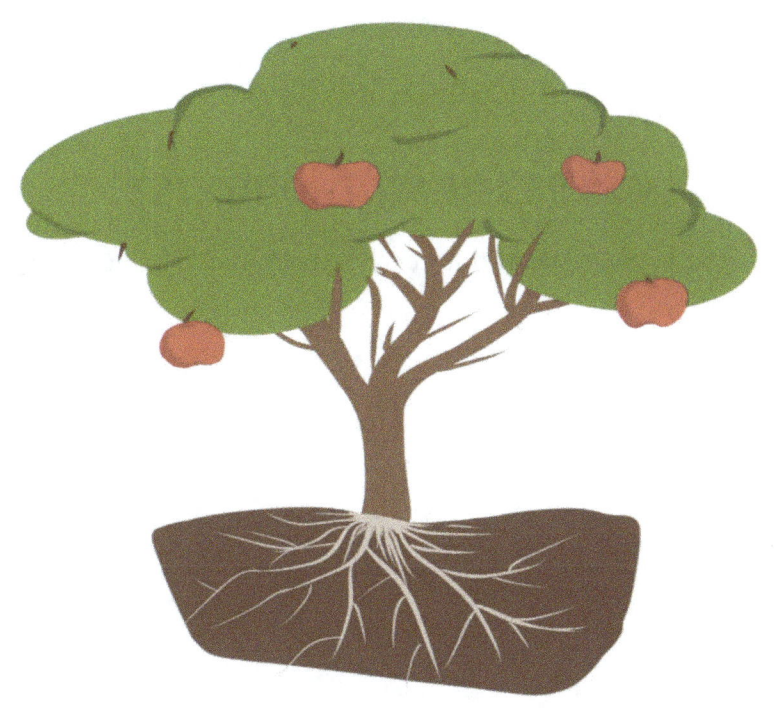

#10 Date:

Right now, I feel _____. I know/do not know (circle one) what triggered this feeling. My triggers as I know them are_____.

_____

_____

_____

WHERE ARE MY THOUGHTS?

My thoughts are focused on my past/present/future (circle one), and they consist of_____.

_____

_____

_____

To Feel Better I Will:

a) Choose the opposite behavior. (Use positive distractions list.)

b) Challenge my thoughts. (Just because I think a thought does not mean it's right!)

c) Limit access to triggers.

d) Silence my inner critic with positive self-talk.

e) Use coping skills. _____

_____

What Are My New Actions?

a) New beliefs and thoughts about the situation:

_____

_____

_____

_____

b) My positive affirmations for today are:

_____

_____

_____

_____

IF YOU DON'T DEAL WITH YOUR PAST, YOUR PAST WILL DEAL WITH YOU!

#11 Date:

Right now, I feel _____. I know/do not know (circle one) what triggered this feeling. My triggers as I know them are_____.

_____

_____

_____

WHERE ARE MY THOUGHTS?

My thoughts are focused on my past/present/future (circle one), and they consist of_____.

_____

_____

_____

To Feel Better I Will:

    a) Choose the opposite behavior. (Use positive distractions list.)

    b) Challenge my thoughts. (Just because I think a thought does not mean it's right!)

    c) Limit access to triggers.

    d) Silence my inner critic with positive self-talk.

    e) Use coping skills. _____

_____

Life Changer Interactive Journal

What Are My New Actions?

a) New beliefs and thoughts about the situation:

___

___

___

___

b) My positive affirmations for today are:

___

___

___

___

WHAT YOU FOCUS ON, YOU EMPOWER!

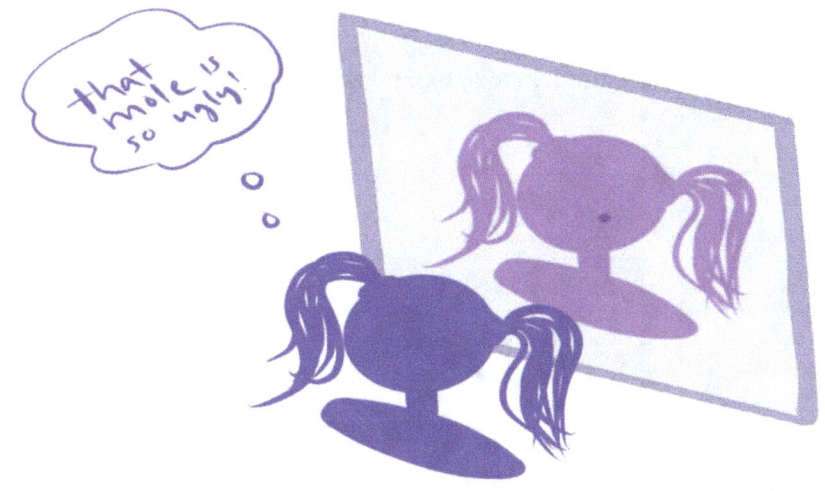

#12 Date:

Right now, I feel _____. I know/do not know (circle one) what triggered this feeling. My triggers as I know them are_____.

_____

_____

_____

_____

WHERE ARE MY THOUGHTS?

My thoughts are focused on my past/present/future (circle one), and they consist of_____.

_____

_____

_____

_____

To Feel Better I Will:

    a) Choose the opposite behavior. (Use positive distractions list.)

    b) Challenge my thoughts. (Just because I think a thought does not mean it's right!)

    c) Limit access to triggers.

    d) Silence my inner critic with positive self-talk.

    e) Use coping skills. _____

_____

What Are My New Actions?

a) New beliefs and thoughts about the situation:

___

___

___

___

b) My positive affirmations for today are:

___

___

___

___

A HOUSE DIVIDED CANNOT STAND! WHO YOU NEED IS YOU!

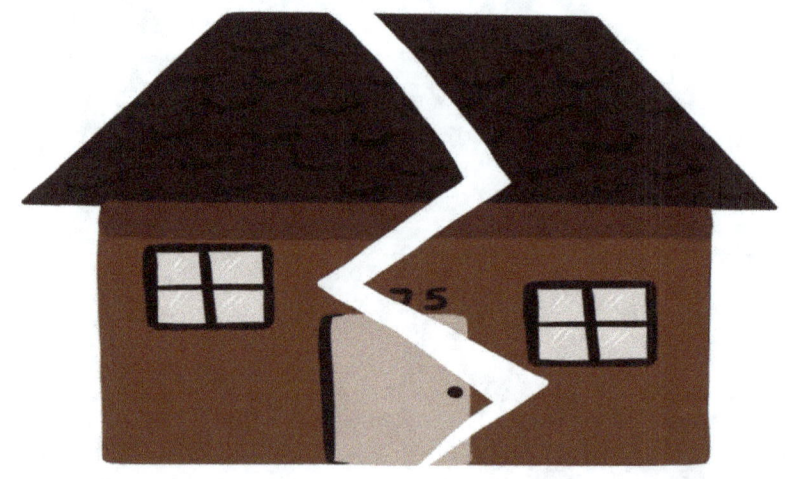

#13 Date:

Right now, I feel _____. I know/do not know (circle one) what triggered this feeling. My triggers as I know them are_____.

_____

_____

_____

_____

WHERE ARE MY THOUGHTS?

My thoughts are focused on my past/present/future (circle one), and they consist of_____.

_____

_____

_____

_____

To Feel Better I Will:

a) Choose the opposite behavior. (Use positive distractions list.)

b) Challenge my thoughts. (Just because I think a thought does not mean it's right!)

c) Limit access to triggers.

d) Silence my inner critic with positive self-talk.

e) Use coping skills. _____

_____

Life Changer Interactive Journal

What Are My New Actions?

    a)   New beliefs and thoughts about the situation:

_____

_____

_____

_____

    b)   My positive affirmations for today are:

_____

_____

_____

_____

FORGIVENESS IS THE KEY TO UNLOCKING THE BALL AND CHAIN!

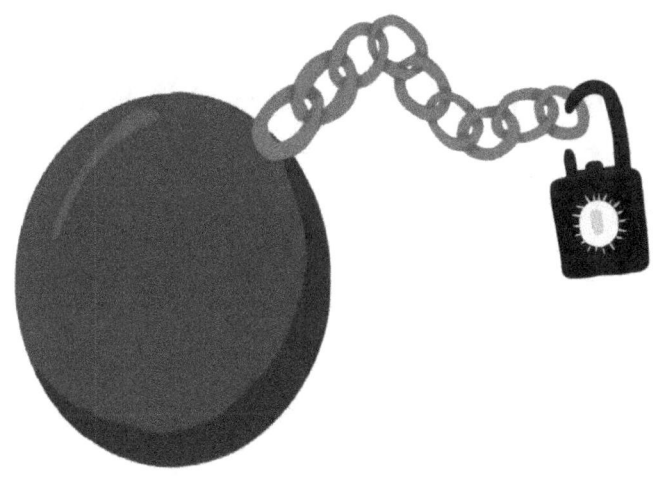

#14 Date:

Right now, I feel _____. I know/do not know (circle one) what triggered this feeling. My triggers as I know them are_____.

_____

_____

_____

WHERE ARE MY THOUGHTS?

My thoughts are focused on my past/present/future (circle one), and they consist of_____.

_____

_____

_____

To Feel Better I Will:

a) Choose the opposite behavior. (Use positive distractions list.)

b) Challenge my thoughts. (Just because I think a thought does not mean it's right!)

c) Limit access to triggers.

d) Silence my inner critic with positive self-talk.

e) Use coping skills. _____

_____

What Are My New Actions?

    a) New beliefs and thoughts about the situation:

___

___

___

___

    b) My positive affirmations for today are:

___

___

___

___

Compare Yourself to Yourself for Measureable Growth!

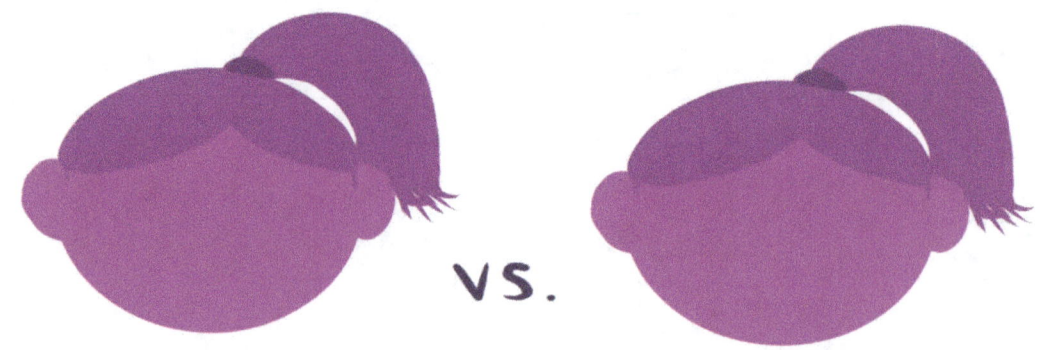

#15 Date:

Right now, I feel _____. I know/do not know (circle one) what triggered this feeling. My triggers as I know them are_____.

_____

_____

_____

_____

WHERE ARE MY THOUGHTS?

My thoughts are focused on my past/present/future (circle one), and they consist of_____.

_____

_____

_____

_____

To Feel Better I Will:

a) Choose the opposite behavior. (Use positive distractions list.)

b) Challenge my thoughts. (Just because I think a thought does not mean it's right!)

c) Limit access to triggers.

d) Silence my inner critic with positive self- talk.

e) Use coping skills. _____

_____

What Are My New Actions?

    a) New beliefs and thoughts about the situation:

    b) My positive affirmations for today are:

CREATING A BETTER VERSION OF SELF DERIVES FROM WITHIN!

#16 Date:

Right now, I feel _____. I know/do not know (circle one) what triggered this feeling. My triggers as I know them are_____.

_____

_____

_____

WHERE ARE MY THOUGHTS?

My thoughts are focused on my past/present/future (circle one), and they consist of_____.

_____

_____

_____

To Feel Better I Will:

a) Choose the opposite behavior. (Use positive distractions list.)

b) Challenge my thoughts. (Just because I think a thought does not mean it's right!)

c) Limit access to triggers.

d) Silence my inner critic with positive self- talk.

e) Use coping skills. _____

_____

What Are My New Actions?

    a)   New beliefs and thoughts about the situation

___

___

___

___

    b)   My positive affirmations for today are:

___

___

___

LOVE YOURSELF UNCONDITIONALLY.
EMBRACE YOUR HIDDEN SELF!

#17 Date:

Right now, I feel _____. I know/do not know (circle one) what triggered this feeling. My triggers as I know them are_____.

_____

_____

_____

WHERE ARE MY THOUGHTS?

My thoughts are focused on my past/present/future (circle one), and they consist of_____.

_____

_____

_____

To Feel Better I Will:

    a) Choose the opposite behavior. (Use positive distractions list.)

    b) Challenge my thoughts. (Just because I think a thought does not mean it's right!)

    c) Limit access to triggers.

    d) Silence my inner critic with positive self-talk.

    e) Use coping skills. _____

_____

Life Changer Interactive Journal

What Are My New Actions?

    a)   New beliefs and thoughts about the situation:

___

___

___

___

    b)   My positive affirmations for today are:

___

___

___

STOP PERPETUATING THE
ABANDONMENT CYCLE.
BE THERE FOR YOU NOW!

#18 Date:

Right now, I feel _____. I know/do not know (circle one) what triggered this feeling. My triggers as I know them are_____.

_____

_____

_____

WHERE ARE MY THOUGHTS?

My thoughts are focused on my past/present/future (circle one), and they consist of_____.

_____

_____

_____

To Feel Better I Will:

a) Choose the opposite behavior. (Use positive distractions list.)

b) Challenge my thoughts. (Just because I think a thought does not mean it's right!)

c) Limit access to triggers.

d) Silence my inner critic with positive self-talk.

e) Use coping skills. _____

_____

What Are My New Actions?

    a)   New beliefs and thoughts about the situation:

___

    b)   My positive affirmations for today are:

DO NOT SAY THINGS TO YOURSELF THAT YOU WOULD NOT WANT OTHER PEOPLE TO SAY TO YOU!

#19 Date:

Right now, I feel _____. I know/do not know (circle one) what triggered this feeling. My triggers as I know them are_____.

_____

_____

_____

WHERE ARE MY THOUGHTS?

My thoughts are focused on my past/present/future (circle one), and they consist of_____.

_____

_____

_____

_____

To Feel Better I Will:

    a) Choose the opposite behavior. (Use positive distractions list.)

    b) Challenge my thoughts. (Just because I think a thought does not mean it's right!)

    c) Limit access to triggers.

    d) Silence my inner critic with positive self-talk.

    e) Use coping skills. _____

_____

Life Changer Interactive Journal

What Are My New Actions?

a) New beliefs and thoughts about the situation:

_____

_____

_____

_____

b) My positive affirmations for today are:

_____

_____

_____

_____

EVERYONE HAS SOME GOOD QUALITIES. WHAT ARE SOME OF YOURS?

1.

2.

3.

4.

5.

#20 Date:

Right now, I feel _____. I know/do not know (circle one) what triggered this feeling. My triggers as I know them are_____.

_____

_____

_____

_____

WHERE ARE MY THOUGHTS?

My thoughts are focused on my past/present/future (circle one), and they consist of_____.

_____

_____

_____

_____

To Feel Better I Will:

    a) Choose the opposite behavior. (Use positive distractions list.)

    b) Challenge my thoughts. (Just because I think a thought does not mean it's right!)

    c) Limit access to triggers.

    d) Silence my inner critic with positive self-talk.

    e) Use coping skills. _____

_____

What Are My New Actions?

    a) New beliefs and thoughts about the situation:

_____

_____

_____

_____

    b) My positive affirmations for today are:

_____

_____

_____

_____

You have paid the "guilt" sentence for too long!

Today is your day of parole!

Live free!

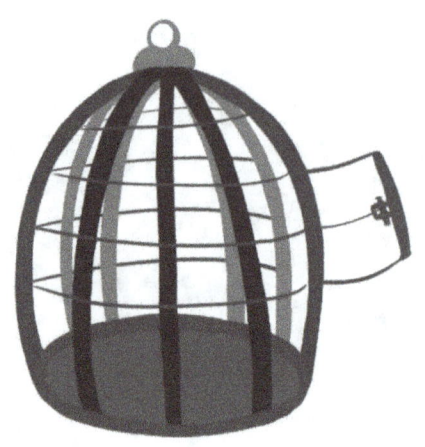

#21 DATE:

Right now, I feel _____. I know/do not know (circle one) what triggered this feeling. My triggers as I know them are_____.

_____

_____

_____

_____

WHERE ARE MY THOUGHTS?

My thoughts are focused on my past/present/future (circle one), and they consist of_____.

_____

_____

_____

_____

To Feel Better I Will:

a) Choose the opposite behavior. (Use positive distractions list.)

b) Challenge my thoughts. (Just because I think a thought does not mean it's right!)

c) Limit access to triggers.

d) Silence my inner critic with positive self-talk.

e) Use coping skills. _____

_____

Life Changer Interactive Journal

What Are My New Actions?

    a)   New beliefs and thoughts about the situation:

___

___

___

___

    b)   My positive affirmations for today are:

___

___

___

___

TODAY IS YOUR DAY OF A TURNAROUND!

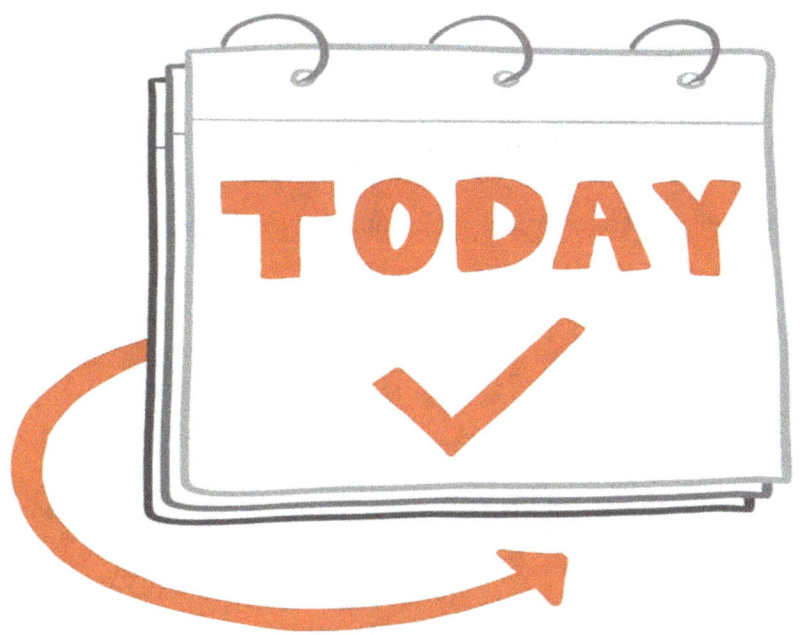

#22 Date:

Right now, I feel _____. I know/do not know (circle one) what triggered this feeling. My triggers as I know them are_____.

_____

_____

_____

WHERE ARE YOUR THOUGHTS?

My thoughts are focused on my past/present/future (circle one), and they consist of_____.

_____

_____

_____

_____

To Feel Better I Will:

a) Choose the opposite behavior. (Use positive distractions list.)

b) Challenge my thoughts. (Just because I think a thought does not mean it's right!)

c) Limit access to triggers.

d) Silence my inner critic with positive self-talk.

e) Use coping skills

What Are My New Actions?

    a) New beliefs and thoughts about the situation:

    _____

    _____

    _____

    _____

    b) My positive affirmations for today are:

    _____

    _____

    _____

    _____

JUST AS CURRENCY IS NOT REDUCED BECAUSE IT HAS BEEN LOST, TOSSED, STEPPED ON, STEPPED OVER, AND TORN; YOUR VALUE IS NOT REDUCED THROUGHOUT YOUR LIFESPAN DUE TO LIFE'S CIRCUMSTANCES! KNOW YOUR WORTH!

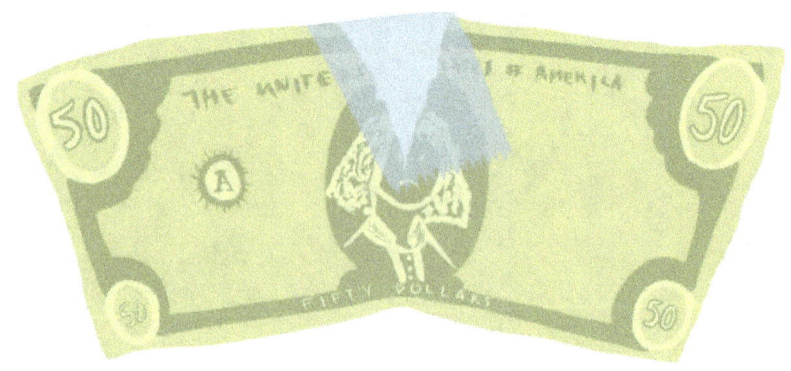

#23 Date:

Right now, I feel _____. I know/do not know (circle one) what triggered this feeling. My triggers as I know them are_____.

_____

_____

_____

_____

WHERE ARE MY THOUGHTS?

My thoughts are focused on my past/present/future (circle one), and they consist of_____.

_____

_____

_____

_____

To Feel Better I Will:

a) Choose the opposite behavior. (Use positive distractions list.)

b) Challenge my thoughts. (Just because I think a thought does not mean it's right!)

c) Limit access to triggers.

d) Silence my inner critic with positive self-talk.

e) Use coping skills. _____

_____

What Are My New Actions?

a) New beliefs and thoughts about the situation:

___

___

___

___

b) My positive affirmations for today are:

___

___

___

___

THIS CIRCUMSTANCE IS ONLY A MOMENT IN TIME. IT IS NOT MY ETERNITY!

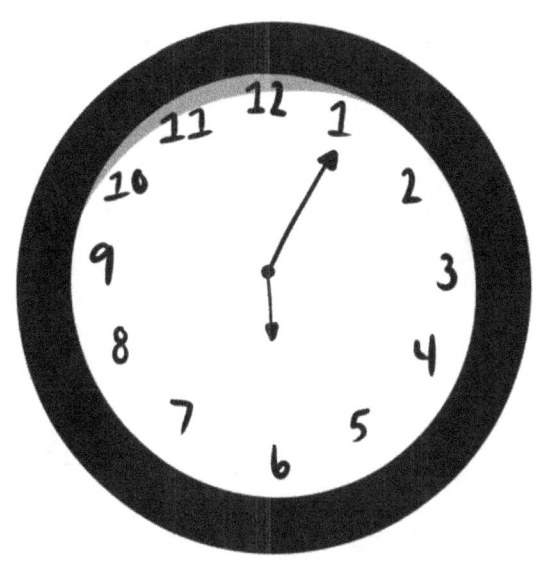

#24 Date:

Right now, I feel _____. I know/do not know (circle one) what triggered this feeling. My triggers as I know them are_____.

_____

_____

_____

WHERE ARE MY THOUGHTS?

My thoughts are focused on my past/present/future (circle one), and they consist of_____.

_____

_____

_____

To Feel Better I Will:

    a) Choose the opposite behavior. (Use positive distractions list.)

    b) Challenge my thoughts. (Just because I think a thought does not mean it's right!)

    c) Limit access to triggers.

    d) Silence my inner critic with positive self-talk.

    e) Use coping skills. _____

_____

What Are My New Actions?

    a) New beliefs and thoughts about the situation:

_____

_____

_____

_____

    b) My positive affirmations for today are:

_____

_____

_____

_____

WHEN EMOTIONS ARE HIGH, SLOW DOWN AND BREATHE. YOU WILL BE ABLE TO THINK A LITTLE CLEARER, AND YOUR CONSEQUENCES WILL BE A LITTLE LIGHTER.

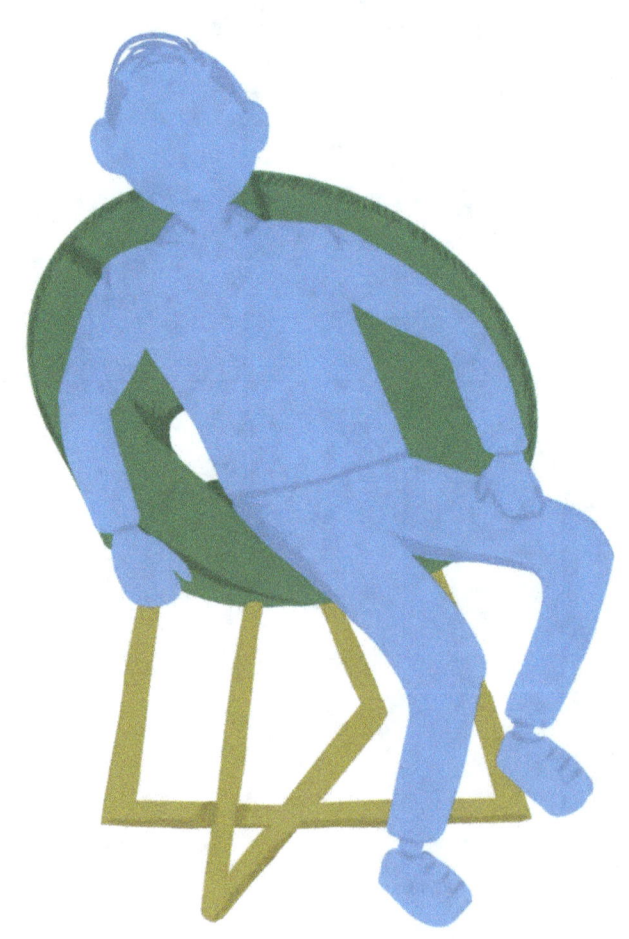

#25 Date:

Right now, I feel _____. I know/do not know (circle one) what triggered this feeling. My triggers as I know them are_____.

_____

_____

_____

WHERE ARE MY THOUGHTS?

My thoughts are focused on my past/present/future (circle one), and they consist of_____.

_____

_____

_____

To Feel Better I Will:

    a) Choose the opposite behavior. (Use positive distractions list.)

    b) Challenge my thoughts. (Just because I think a thought does not mean it's right!)

    c) Limit access to triggers.

    d) Silence my inner critic with positive self-talk.

    e) Use coping skills. _____

_____

Life Changer Interactive Journal

What Are My New Actions?

    a)   New beliefs and thoughts about the situation:

___

___

___

___

    b)   My positive affirmations for today are:

___

___

___

___

CHANGE IS HARD BUT DOABLE!

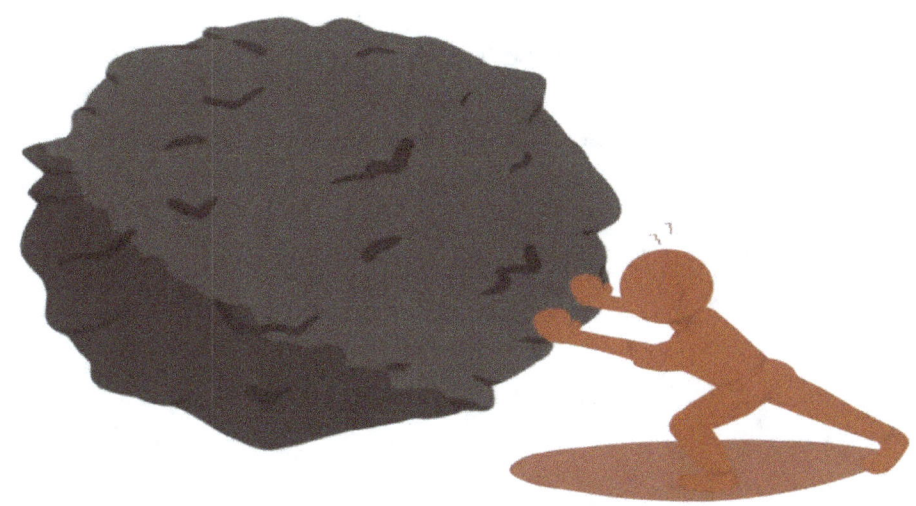

#26 Date:

Right now, I feel _____. I know/do not know (circle one) what triggered this feeling. My triggers as I know them are_____.

_____

_____

_____

WHERE ARE MY THOUGHTS?

My thoughts are focused on my past/present/future (circle one), and they consist of_____.

_____

_____

_____

To Feel Better I Will:

a) Choose the opposite behavior. (Use positive distractions list.)

b) Challenge my thoughts. (Just because I think a thought does not mean it is right!)

c) Limit access to triggers.

d) Silence my inner critic with positive self-talk.

e) Use coping skills. _____

_____

What Are My New Actions?

    a)   New beliefs and thoughts about the situation:

___

___

___

___

    b)   My positive affirmations for today are:

___

___

___

___

JUST BECAUSE YOU THINK A THOUGHT, DOES NOT MEAN THE THOUGHT IS RIGHT!

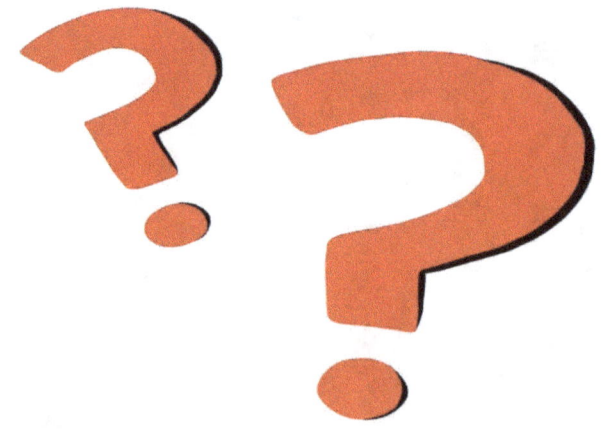

#27 Date:

Right now, I feel _____. I know/do not know (circle one) what triggered this feeling. My triggers as I know them are_____.

_____

_____

_____

_____

WHERE ARE MY THOUGHTS?

My thoughts are focused on my past/present/future (circle one), and they consist of_____.

_____

_____

_____

_____

To Feel Better I Will:

    a) Choose the opposite behavior. (Use positive distractions list.)

    b) Challenge my thoughts. (Just because I think a thought does not mean it's right!)

    c) Limit access to triggers.

    d) Silence my inner critic with positive self-talk.

    e) Use coping skills. _____

_____

Life Changer Interactive Journal

What Are My New Actions?

    a)   New beliefs and thoughts about the situation:

___

___

___

___

    b)   My positive affirmations for today are:

___

___

___

___

AWARENESS ILLUMINATES YOUR PATH

#28 Date:

Right now, I feel _____. I know/do not know (circle one) what triggered this feeling. My triggers as I know them are_____.

_____

_____

_____

WHERE ARE MY THOUGHTS?

My thoughts are focused on my past/present/future (circle one), and they consist of_____.

_____

_____

_____

To Feel Better I Will:

a) Choose the opposite behavior. (Use positive distractions list.)

b) Challenge my thoughts. (Just because I think a thought does not mean it's right!)

c) Limit access to triggers.

d) Silence my inner critic with positive self-talk.

e) Use coping skills. _____

_____

What Are My New Actions?

    a) New beliefs and thoughts about the situation:

_____

_____

_____

_____

    b) My positive affirmations for today are:

_____

_____

_____

_____

WHATEVER YOU DO, DO IT
WHOLEHEARTEDLY WITH PASSION.
BE THE EXPERIENCE!

#29 Date:

Right now, I feel _____. I know/do not know (circle one) what triggered this feeling. My triggers as I know them are_____.

_____

_____

_____

_____

WHERE ARE MY THOUGHTS?

My thoughts are focused on my past/present/future (circle one), and they consist of_____.

_____

_____

_____

_____

To Feel Better I Will:

a) Choose the opposite behavior. (Use positive distractions list.)

b) Challenge my thoughts. (Just because I think a thought does not mean it's right!)

c) Limit access to triggers.

d) Silence my inner critic with positive self-talk.

e) Use coping skills. _____

_____

Life Changer Interactive Journal

What Are My New Actions?

a) New beliefs and thoughts about the situation:

_____

_____

_____

_____

b) My positive affirmations for today are:

_____

_____

_____

_____

**ACCEPT IT. SIT WITH IT.
KEEP IT MOVING!
ASK!**

#30 Date:

Right now, I feel _____. I know/do not know (circle one) what triggered this feeling. My triggers as I know them are_____.

_____

_____

_____

_____

WHERE ARE MY THOUGHTS?

My thoughts are focused on my past/present/future (circle one), and they consist of_____.

_____

_____

_____

_____

To Feel Better I Will:

    a) Choose the opposite behavior. (Use positive distractions list.)

    b) Challenge my thoughts. (Just because I think a thought does not mean it's right!)

    c) Limit access to triggers.

    d) Silence my inner critic with positive self-talk.

    e) Use coping skills. _____

_____

What Are My New Actions?

    a) New beliefs and thoughts about the situation:

    b) My positive affirmations for today are:

RAIN IS YOUR OPPORTUNITY TO GROW, BE NURTURED, AND BLOOM!

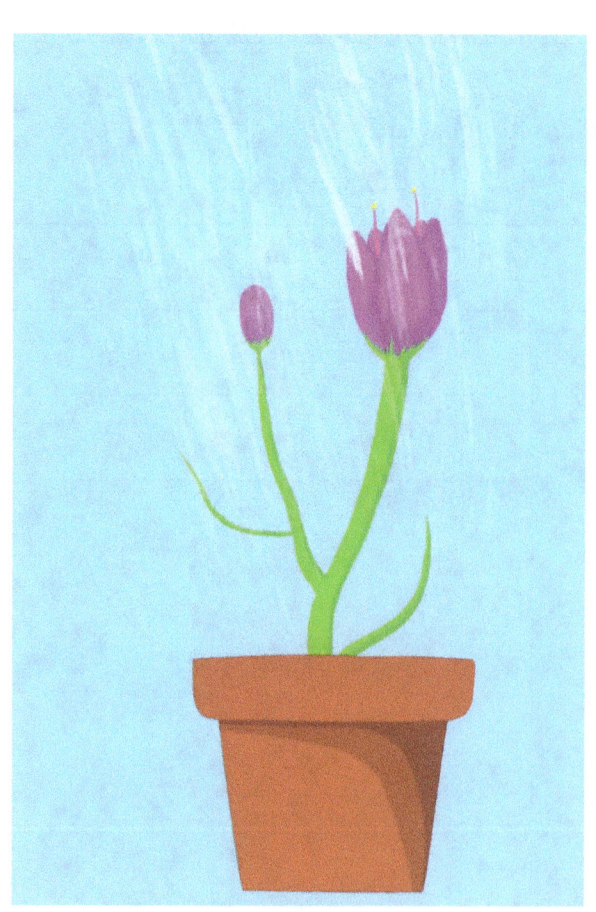

#31 Date:

Right now, I feel _____. I know/do not know (circle one) what triggered this feeling. My triggers as I know them are_____.

_____

_____

_____

_____

WHERE ARE MY THOUGHTS?

My thoughts are focused on my past/present/future (circle one), and they consist of_____.

_____

_____

_____

_____

To Feel Better I Will:

    a) Choose the opposite behavior. (Use positive distractions list.)

    b) Challenge my thoughts. (Just because I think a thought does not mean it's right!)

    c) Limit access to triggers.

    d) Silence my inner critic with positive self-talk.

    e) Use coping skills. _____

_____

Life Changer Interactive Journal

What Are My New Actions?

    a)   New beliefs and thoughts about the situation:

    b)   My positive affirmations for today are:

YOU CAN HAVE A DIAGNOSIS,
AS LONG AS THE DIAGNOSIS
DOES NOT HAVE YOU!

#32 Date:

Right now, I feel _____. I know/do not know (circle one) what triggered this feeling. My triggers as I know them are _____.

_____

_____

_____

WHERE ARE MY THOUGHTS?

My thoughts are focused on my past/present/future (circle one), and they consist of _____.

_____

_____

_____

To Feel Better I Will:

a) Choose the opposite behavior. (Use positive distractions list.)

b) Challenge my thoughts. (Just because I think a thought does not mean it's right!)

c) Limit access to triggers.

d) Silence my inner critic with positive self-talk.

e) Use coping skills. _____

_____

What Are My New Actions?

    a)   New beliefs and thoughts about the situation:

_____

_____

_____

_____

    b)   My positive affirmations for today are:

_____

_____

_____

_____

DO NOT DWELL IN THE CAMP OF NEGATIVITY!

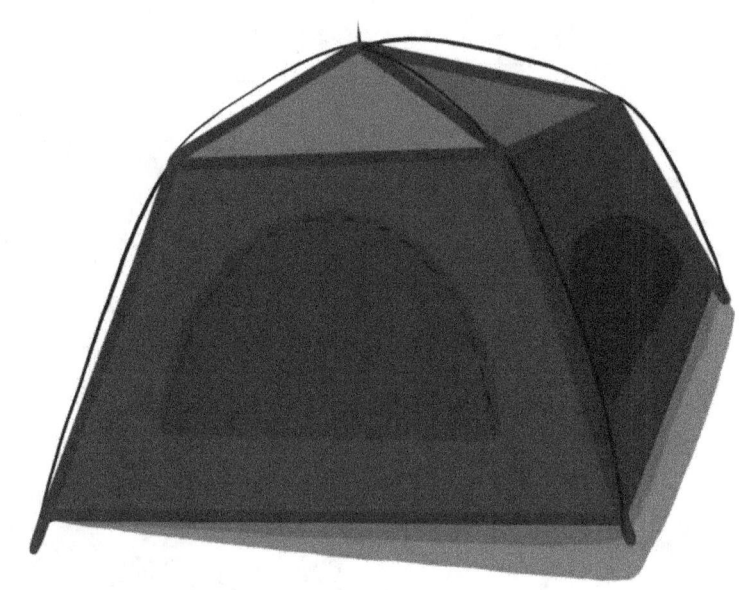

#33 Date:

Right now, I feel _____. I know/do not know (circle one) what triggered this feeling. My triggers as I know them are_____.

_____

_____

_____

_____

WHERE ARE MY THOUGHTS?

My thoughts are focused on my past/present/future (circle one), and they consist of_____.

_____

_____

_____

_____

To Feel Better I Will:

    a) Choose the opposite behavior. (Use positive distractions list.)

    b) Challenge my thoughts. (Just because I think a thought does not mean it's right!)

    c) Limit access to triggers.

    d) Silence my inner critic with positive self-talk.

    e) Use coping skills. _____

Life Changer Interactive Journal

What Are My New Actions?

a) New beliefs and thoughts about the situation:

___

___

___

___

b) My positive affirmations for today are:

___

___

___

___

PRESS PAST YOUR PAIN!

#34 Date:

Right now, I feel _____. I know/do not know (circle one) what triggered this feeling. My triggers as I know them are_____.

_____

_____

_____

WHERE ARE MY THOUGHTS?

My thoughts are focused on my past/present/future (circle one), and they consist of_____.

_____

_____

_____

To Feel Better I Will:

    a) Choose the opposite behavior. (Use positive distractions list.)

    b) Challenge my thoughts. (Just because I think a thought does not mean it's right!)

    c) Limit access to triggers.

    d) Silence my inner critic with positive self-talk.

    e) Use coping skills. _____

_____

What Are My New Actions?

    a) New beliefs and thoughts about the situation:

_____

_____

_____

_____

    b) My positive affirmations for today are:

_____

_____

_____

_____

FORGIVENESS BENEFITS ME!

#35 Date:

Right now, I feel _____. I know/do not know (circle one) what triggered this feeling. My triggers as I know them are_____.

_____

_____

_____

_____

WHERE ARE MY THOUGHTS?

My thoughts are focused on my past/present/future (circle one), and they consist of_____.

_____

_____

_____

_____

To Feel Better I Will:

a) Choose the opposite behavior. (Use positive distractions list.)

b) Challenge my thoughts. (Just because I think a thought does not mean it's right!)

c) Limit access to triggers.

d) Silence my inner critic with positive self-talk.

e) Use coping skills. _____

_____

What Are My New Actions?

a) New beliefs and thoughts about the situation:

_____

_____

_____

_____

b) My positive affirmations for today are:

_____

_____

_____

_____

Validate your emotions.
Don't wait on others to validate
them for you!

#36 Date:

Right now, I feel _____. I know/do not know (circle one) what triggered this feeling. My triggers as I know them are_____.

_____

_____

_____

WHERE ARE YOUR THOUGHTS?

My thoughts are focused on my past/present/future (circle one), and they consist of_____.

_____

_____

_____

To Feel Better I Will:

    a) Choose the opposite behavior. (Use positive distractions list.)

    b) Challenge my thoughts. (Just because I think a thought does not mean it's right!)

    c) Limit access to triggers.

    d) Silence my inner critic with positive self-talk.

    e) Use coping skills. _____

_____

What Are My New Actions?

    a) New beliefs and thoughts about the situation:

    b) My positive affirmations for today are:

SECRET PAIN PERPETUATES A
DESTRUCTIVE CYCLE.
USE YOUR VOICE!

#37 Date:

Right now, I feel _____. I know/do not know (circle one) what triggered this feeling. My triggers as I know them are_____.

_____

_____

_____

_____

WHERE ARE MY THOUGHTS?

My thoughts are focused on my past/present/future (circle one), and they consist of_____.

_____

_____

_____

_____

To Feel Better I Will:

a) Choose the opposite behavior. (Use positive distractions list.)

b) Challenge my thoughts. (Just because I think a thought does not mean it's right!)

c) Limit access to triggers.

d) Silence my inner critic with positive self-talk.

e) Use coping skills. _____

_____

Life Changer Interactive Journal

What Are My New Actions?

a) New beliefs and thoughts about the situation:

___

___

___

___

b) My positive affirmations for today are:

___

___

___

___

THE JOURNEY TOWARDS YOUR GREATER SELF ENTAILS BOTH HILLS AND VALLEYS.

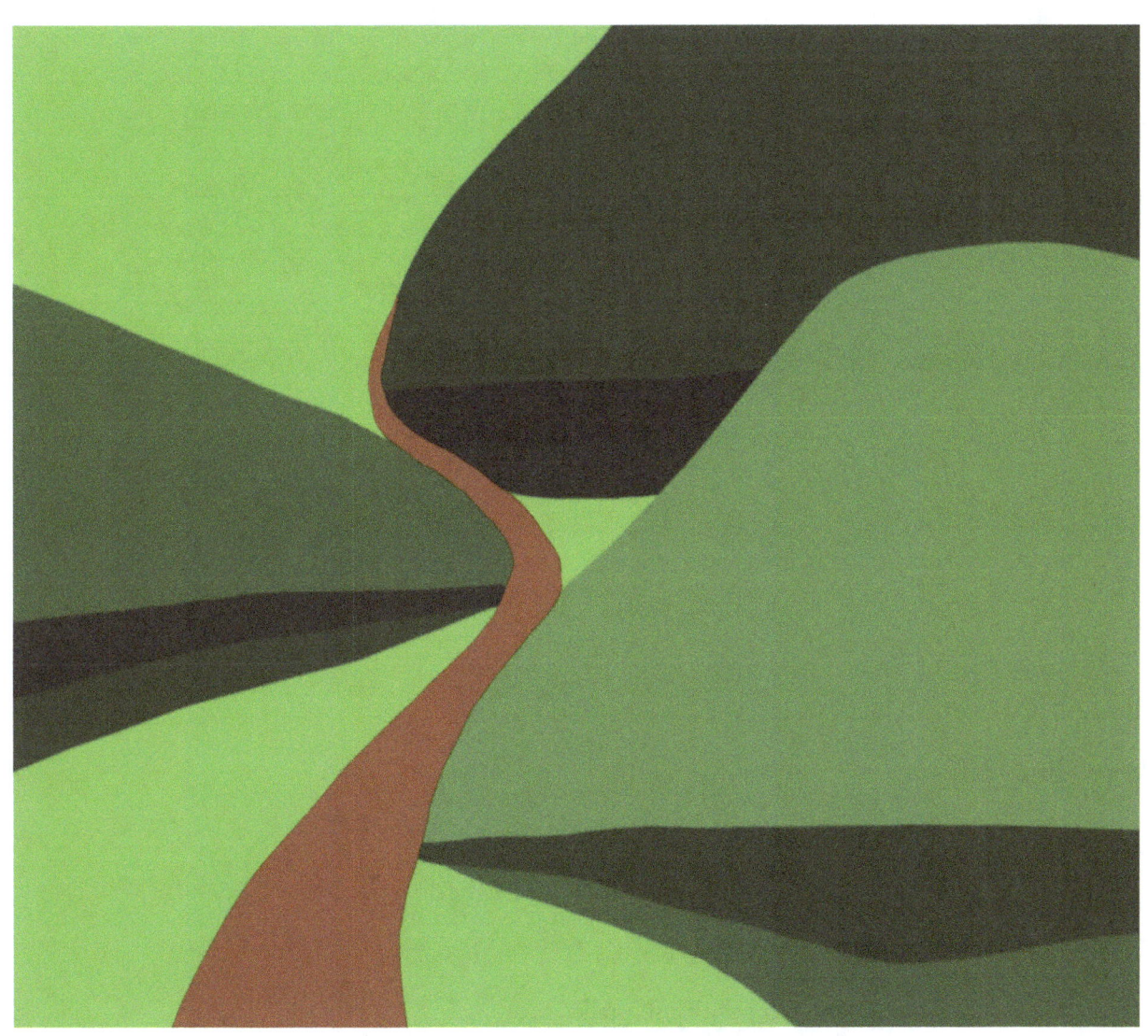

#38 Date:

Right now, I feel _____. I know/do not know (circle one) what triggered this feeling. My triggers as I know them are_____.

_____

_____

_____

_____

WHERE ARE MY THOUGHTS?

My thoughts are focused on my past/present/future (circle one), and they consist of_____.

_____

_____

_____

_____

To Feel Better I Will:

    a) Choose the opposite behavior. (Use positive distractions list.)

    b) Challenge my thoughts. (Just because I think a thought does not mean it's right!)

    c) Limit access to triggers.

    d) Silence my inner critic with positive self-talk.

    e) Use coping skills. _____

_____

What Are My New Actions?

a) New beliefs and thoughts about the situation:

b) My positive affirmations for today are:

BEING FREE REQUIRES FORGIVENESS
OF SELF AND OTHERS.
CHOOSE FREEDOM!

#39 Date:

Right now, I feel _____. I know/do not know (circle one) what triggered this feeling. My triggers as I know them are_____.

_____

_____

_____

_____

WHERE ARE MY THOUGHTS?

My thoughts are focused on my past/present/future (circle one), and they consist of_____.

_____

_____

_____

_____

To Feel Better I Will:

a) Choose the opposite behavior. (Use positive distractions list.)

b) Challenge my thoughts. (Just because I think a thought does not mean it's right!)

c) Limit access to triggers.

d) Silence my inner critic with positive self-talk.

e) Use coping skills. _____

_____

What Are My New Actions?

a) New beliefs and thoughts about the situation:

___

___

___

___

b) My positive affirmations for today are:

___

___

___

___

THOUGHTS = FEELINGS
FEELINGS = BEHAVIORS
BEHAVIORS = CONSEQUENCES

#40 Date:

Right now, I feel _____. I know/do not know (circle one) what triggered this feeling. My triggers as I know them are_____.

_____

_____

_____

WHERE ARE MY THOUGHTS?

My thoughts are focused on my past/present/future (circle one), and they consist of_____.

_____

_____

_____

To Feel Better I Will:

a) Choose the opposite behavior. (Use positive distractions list.)

b) Challenge my thoughts. (Just because I think a thought does not mean it's right!)

c) Limit access to triggers.

d) Silence my inner critic with positive self-talk.

e) Use coping skills. _____

_____

What Are My New Actions?

    a)   New beliefs and thoughts about the situation:

___

___

___

___

    b)   My positive affirmations for today are:

___

___

___

___

Life Changer Interactive Journal

IS YOUR DESIRE TO CHANGE GREATER THAN YOUR DESIRE TO REMAIN THE SAME?

#41 Date:

Right now, I feel _____. I know/do not know (circle one) what triggered this feeling. My triggers as I know them are_____.

_____

_____

_____

WHERE ARE MY THOUGHTS?

My thoughts are focused on my past/present/future (circle one), and they consist of_____.

_____

_____

_____

To Feel Better I Will:

a) Choose the opposite behavior. (Use positive distractions list.)

b) Challenge my thoughts. (Just because I think a thought does not mean it's right!)

c) Limit access to triggers.

d) Silence my inner critic with positive self-talk.

e) Use coping skills. _____

_____

What Are My New Actions?

    a)   New beliefs and thoughts about the situation:

_____

_____

_____

_____

    b)   My positive affirmations for today are:

_____

_____

_____

_____

You are the master architect of your life! Are you constructive or destructive?

#42 Date:

Right now, I feel _____. I know/do not know (circle one) what triggered this feeling. My triggers as I know them are_____.

_____

_____

_____

WHERE ARE MY THOUGHTS?

My thoughts are focused on my past/present/future (circle one), and they consist of_____.

_____

_____

_____

To Feel Better I Will:

    a) Choose the opposite behavior. (Use positive distractions list.)

    b) Challenge my thoughts. (Just because I think a thought does not mean it's right!)

    c) Limit access to triggers.

    d) Silence my inner critic with positive self-talk.

    e) Use coping skills. _____

_____

What Are My New Actions?

a) New beliefs and thoughts about the situation:

b) My positive affirmations for today are:

EMOTIONAL HEALING REQUIRES VULNERABILITY.

#43 Date:

Right now, I feel _____. I know/do not know (circle one) what triggered this feeling. My triggers as I know them are_____.

_____

_____

_____

WHERE ARE MY THOUGHTS?

My thoughts are focused on my past/present/future (circle one), and they consist of_____.

_____

_____

_____

To Feel Better I Will:

a) Choose the opposite behavior. (Use positive distractions list.)

b) Challenge my thoughts. (Just because I think a thought does not mean it's right!)

c) Limit access to triggers.

d) Silence my inner critic with positive self-talk.

e) Use coping skills. _____

Life Changer Interactive Journal

What Are My New Actions?

a) New beliefs and thoughts about the situation:

_____

_____

_____

_____

b) My positive affirmations for today are:

_____

_____

_____

_____

AS LONG AS YOU ARE INHALING AND EXHALING, YOU CAN BEGIN AGAIN.

#44 Date:

Right now, I feel _____. I know/do not know (circle one) what triggered this feeling. My triggers as I know them are_____.

_____

_____

_____

WHERE ARE MY THOUGHTS?

My thoughts are focused on my past/present/future (circle one), and they consist of_____.

_____

_____

_____

To Feel Better I Will:

a) Choose the opposite behavior. (Use positive distractions list.)

b) Challenge my thoughts. (Just because I think a thought does not mean it's right!)

c) Limit access to triggers.

d) Silence my inner critic with positive self-talk.

e) Use coping skills. _____

_____

What Are My New Actions?

a) New beliefs and thoughts about the situation:

_____

_____

_____

_____

b) My positive affirmations for today are:

_____

_____

_____

_____

What others think about you is not as important as what you think about yourself!

#45 Date:

Right now, I feel _____. I know/do not know (circle one) what triggered this feeling. My triggers as I know them are_____.

_____

_____

_____

_____

WHERE ARE MY THOUGHTS?

My thoughts are focused on my past/present/future (circle one), and they consist of_____.

_____

_____

_____

_____

To Feel Better I Will:

    a) Choose the opposite behavior. (Use positive distractions list.)

    b) Challenge my thoughts. (Just because I think a thought does not mean it's right!)

    c) Limit access to triggers.

    d) Silence my inner critic with positive self-talk.

    e) Use coping skills. _____

_____

Life Changer Interactive Journal

What Are My New Actions?

a) New beliefs and thoughts about the situation:

_____

_____

_____

_____

b) My positive affirmations for today are:

_____

_____

_____

_____

IT'S OK TO HAVE ANGER WHEN ANGER DOES NOT HAVE YOU!

#46 Date:

Right now, I feel _____. I know/do not know (circle one) what triggered this feeling. My triggers as I know them are_____.

_____

_____

_____

WHERE ARE MY THOUGHTS?

My thoughts are focused on my past/present/future (circle one), and they consist of_____.

_____

_____

_____

To Feel Better I Will:

a) Choose the opposite behavior. (Use positive distractions list.)

b) Challenge my thoughts. (Just because I think a thought does not mean it's right!)

c) Limit access to triggers.

d) Silence my inner critic with positive self-talk.

e) Use coping skills. _____

What Are My New Actions?

    a) New beliefs and thoughts about the situation:

_____

_____

_____

_____

    b) My positive affirmations for today are:

_____

_____

_____

_____

VVR!

Value, Validate, and Respect Yourself!

#47 Date:

Right now, I feel _____. I know/do not know (circle one) what triggered this feeling. My triggers as I know them are_____.

_____

_____

_____

WHERE ARE MY THOUGHTS?

My thoughts are focused on my past/present/future (circle one), and they consist of_____.

_____

_____

_____

To Feel Better I Will:

   a) Choose the opposite behavior. (Use positive distractions list.)

   b) Challenge my thoughts. (Just because I think a thought does not mean it's right!)

   c) Limit access to triggers.

   d) Silence my inner critic with positive self-talk.

   e) Use coping skills. _____

_____

What Are My New Actions?

    a) New beliefs and thoughts about the situation:

___

___

___

___

    b) My positive affirmations for today are:

___

___

___

___

WHOLENESS BEGINS WITHIN!

#48 Date:

Right now, I feel _____. I know/do not know (circle one) what triggered this feeling. My triggers as I know them are_____.

_____

_____

_____

_____

WHERE ARE MY THOUGHTS?

My thoughts are focused on my past/present/future (circle one), and they consist of_____.

_____

_____

_____

_____

To Feel Better I Will:

a) Choose the opposite behavior. (Use positive distractions list.)

b) Challenge my thoughts. (Just because I think a thought does not mean it's right!)

c) Limit access to triggers.

d) Silence my inner critic with positive self-talk.

e) Use coping skills. _____

_____

What Are My New Actions?

    a) New beliefs and thoughts about the situation:

___

___

___

___

    b) My positive affirmations for today are:

___

___

___

___

TAKE TIME TODAY TO BREATHE DEEPLY! EXERCISE:

INHALE THROUGH THE NOSE FOR A COUNT OF FOUR.

HOLD FOR A COUNT OF SEVEN.

EXHALE SLOWLY FOR A COUNT OF EIGHT.

FOUR ROUNDS AT A TIME.

#49 Date:

Right now, I feel _____. I know/do not know (circle one) what triggered this feeling. My triggers as I know them are_____.

_____

_____

_____

WHERE ARE MY THOUGHTS?

My thoughts are focused on my past/present/future (circle one), and they consist of_____.

_____

_____

_____

To Feel Better I Will:

    a) Choose the opposite behavior. (Use positive distractions list.)

    b) Challenge my thoughts. (Just because I think a thought does not mean it's right!)

    c) Limit access to triggers.

    d) Silence my inner critic with positive self-talk.

    e) Use coping skills. _____

_____

Life Changer Interactive Journal

What Are My New Actions?

a) New beliefs and thoughts about the situation:

_____

_____

_____

_____

b) My positive affirmations for today are:

_____

_____

_____

_____

What Are You Grateful For?

1.

2.

3.

4.

5.

#50 Date:

Right now, I feel _____. I know/do not know (circle one) what triggered this feeling. My triggers as I know them are_____.

_____

_____

_____

WHERE ARE MY THOUGHTS?

My thoughts are focused on my past/present/future (circle one), and they consist of_____.

_____

_____

_____

To Feel Better I Will:

    a) Choose the opposite behavior. (Use positive distractions list.)

    b) Challenge my thoughts. (Just because I think a thought does not mean it's right!)

    c) Limit access to triggers.

    d) Silence my inner critic with positive self-talk.

    e) Use coping skills. _____

What Are My New Actions?

    a) New beliefs and thoughts about the situation:

    _____

    _____

    _____

    _____

    b) My positive affirmations for today are:

    _____

    _____

    _____

    _____

GROUND YOURSELF WITH MINDFULNESS!

1. What are 5 things you see?

    a._____

    b._____

    c._____

    d._____

    e._____

2. What are 4 things you hear?

    a._____

    b._____

    c._____

    d._____

3. What are 3 things you can feel?

   a._____

   b._____

   c._____

4. What are 2 things your smell?

   a._____

   b._____

5. What is 1 thing you taste? (gum, mints, etc.)

   a._____

#51 Date:

Right now, I feel _____. I know/do not know (circle one) what triggered this feeling. My triggers as I know them are_____.

_____

_____

_____

_____

WHERE ARE MY THOUGHTS?

My thoughts are focused on my past/present/future (circle one), and they consist of_____.

_____

_____

_____

_____

To Feel Better I Will:

a) Choose the opposite behavior. (Use positive distractions list.)

b) Challenge my thoughts. (Just because I think a thought does not mean it's right!)

c) Limit access to triggers.

d) Silence my inner critic with positive self-talk.

e) Use coping skills. _____

_____

What Are My New Actions?

    a) New beliefs and thoughts about the situation:

_____

_____

_____

_____

    b) My positive affirmations for today are:

_____

_____

_____

_____

THE VOICE OF YOUR INNER CRITIC HAS A BIG MOUTH!
SILENCE ITS VOICE WITH LOVE!

#52 Date:

Right now, I feel _____. I know/do not know (circle one) what triggered this feeling. My triggers as I know them are_____.

_____

_____

_____

_____

WHERE ARE MY THOUGHTS?

My thoughts are focused on my past/present/future (circle one), and they consist of_____.

_____

_____

_____

_____

To Feel Better I Will:

    a) Choose the opposite behavior. (Use positive distractions list.)

    b) Challenge my thoughts. (Just because I think a thought does not mean it's right!)

    c) Limit access to triggers.

    d) Silence my inner critic with positive self-talk.

    e) Use coping skills. _____

_____

What Are My New Actions?

    a) New beliefs and thoughts about the situation:

___

___

___

___

    b) My positive affirmations for today are:

___

___

___

___

ONE OF THE GREATEST RELATIONSHIPS YOU CAN HAVE IS THE RELATIONSHIP WITH YOURSELF!

#53 Date:

Right now, I feel _____. I know/do not know (circle one) what triggered this feeling. My triggers as I know them are_____.

_____

_____

_____

_____

WHERE ARE MY THOUGHTS?

My thoughts are focused on my past/present/future (circle one), and they consist of_____.

_____

_____

_____

_____

To Feel Better I Will:

    a) Choose the opposite behavior. (Use positive distractions list.)

    b) Challenge my thoughts. (Just because I think a thought does not mean it's right!)

    c) Limit access to triggers.

    d) Silence my inner critic with positive self-talk.

    e) Use coping skills. _____

_____

What Are My New Actions?

    a) New beliefs and thoughts about the situation:

_____

_____

_____

_____

    b) My positive affirmations for today are:

_____

_____

_____

_____

FOOD IS MOOD AND MEDICINE.
WHAT ARE YOU EATING?

#54 Date:

Right now, I feel _____. I know/do not know (circle one) what triggered this feeling. My triggers as I know them are_____.

_____

_____

_____

WHERE ARE MY THOUGHTS?

My thoughts are focused on my past/present/future (circle one), and they consist of_____.

_____

_____

_____

To Feel Better I Will:

    a) Choose the opposite behavior. (Use positive distractions list.)

    b) Challenge my thoughts. (Just because I think a thought does not mean it's right!)

    c) Limit access to triggers.

    d) Silence my inner critic with positive self-talk.

    e) Use coping skills. _____

_____

What Are My New Actions?

a) New beliefs and thoughts about the situation:

_____

_____

_____

_____

b) My positive affirmations for today are:

_____

_____

_____

_____

TO MOVE FORWARD, RADICALLY ACCEPT YOUR CURRENT CIRCUMSTANCE!

#55 Date:

Right now, I feel _____. I know/do not know (circle one) what triggered this feeling. My triggers as I know them are_____.

_____

_____

_____

WHERE ARE MY THOUGHTS?

My thoughts are focused on my past/present/future (circle one), and they consist of_____.

_____

_____

_____

To Feel Better I Will:

    a) Choose the opposite behavior. (Use positive distractions list.)

    b) Challenge my thoughts. (Just because I think a thought does not mean it's right!)

    c) Limit access to triggers.

    d) Silence my inner critic with positive self-talk.

    e) Use coping skills. _____

_____

What Are My New Actions?

    a) New beliefs and thoughts about the situation:

    _____

    _____

    _____

    _____

    b) My positive affirmations for today are:

    _____

    _____

    _____

    _____

Allow Pain to Push You into Your Purpose!

#56 Date:

Right now, I feel _____. I know/do not know (circle one) what triggered this feeling. My triggers as I know them are_____.

_____

_____

_____

_____

WHERE ARE MY THOUGHTS?

My thoughts are focused on my past/present/future (circle one), and they consist of_____.

_____

_____

_____

_____

To Feel Better I Will:

   a) Choose the opposite behavior. (Use positive distractions list.)

   b) Challenge my thoughts. (Just because I think a thought does not mean it's right!)

   c) Limit access to triggers.

   d) Silence my inner critic with positive self-talk.

   e) Use coping skills. _____

_____

What Are My New Actions?

    a) New beliefs and thoughts about the situation:

    _____

    _____

    _____

    _____

    b) My positive affirmations for today are:

    _____

    _____

    _____

    _____

AS PLANTS NEED DIRT TO GROW, SO DO WE.
DO NOT DESPISE YOUR DIRTY PLACES!

#57 Date:

Right now, I feel _____. I know/do not know (circle one) what triggered this feeling. My triggers as I know them are_____.

_____

_____

_____

_____

WHERE ARE MY THOUGHTS?

My thoughts are focused on my past/present/future (circle one), and they consist of_____.

_____

_____

_____

_____

To Feel Better I Will:

a) Choose the opposite behavior. (Use positive distractions list.)

b) Challenge my thoughts. (Just because I think a thought does not mean it's right!)

c) Limit access to triggers.

d) Silence my inner critic with positive self-talk.

e) Use coping skills. _____

_____

What Are My New Actions?

    a) New beliefs and thoughts about the situation:

    b) My positive affirmations for today are:

PLANT SEEDS OF FAITH, AND HOPE IN YOUR SUBCONSCIOUS GARDEN

#58 Date:

Right now, I feel _____. I know/do not know (circle one) what triggered this feeling. My triggers as I know them are_____.

_____

_____

_____

WHERE ARE MY THOUGHTS?

My thoughts are focused on my past/present/future (circle one), and they consist of_____.

_____

_____

_____

To Feel Better I Will:

    a) Choose the opposite behavior. (Use positive distractions list.)

    b) Challenge my thoughts. (Just because I think a thought does not mean it's right!)

    c) Limit access to triggers.

    d) Silence my inner critic with positive self-talk.

    e) Use coping skills. _____

_____

Life Changer Interactive Journal

What Are My New Actions?

a) New beliefs and thoughts about the situation:

b) My positive affirmations for today are:

FOLLOWING YOUR NEGATIVE EMOTIONS WILL TAKE YOU DOWN A DESTRUCTIVE PATH!

#59 Date:

Right now, I feel _____. I know/do not know (circle one) what triggered this feeling. My triggers as I know them are_____.

_____

_____

_____

WHERE ARE MY THOUGHTS?

My thoughts are focused on my past/present/future (circle one), and they consist of_____.

_____

_____

_____

To Feel Better I Will:

a) Choose the opposite behavior. (Use positive distractions list.)

b) Challenge my thoughts. (Just because I think a thought does not mean it's right!)

c) Limit access to triggers.

d) Silence my inner critic with positive self-talk.

e) Use coping skills. _____

What Are My New Actions?

   a) New beliefs and thoughts about the situation:

   _____

   _____

   _____

   _____

   b) My positive affirmations for today are:

   _____

   _____

   _____

   _____

PAIN IS THE MASTER TEACHER! WHAT LESSONS HAVE YOU LEARNED?

#60 Date:

Right now, I feel _____. I know/do not know (circle one) what triggered this feeling. My triggers as I know them are_____.

_____

_____

_____

WHERE ARE MY THOUGHTS?

My thoughts are focused on my past/present/future (circle one), and they consist of_____.

_____

_____

_____

To Feel Better I Will:

a) Choose the opposite behavior. (Use positive distractions list.)

b) Challenge my thoughts. (Just because I think a thought does not mean it's right!)

c) Limit access to triggers.

d) Silence my inner critic with positive self-talk.

e) Use coping skills. _____

Life Changer Interactive Journal

What Are My New Actions?

a) New beliefs and thoughts about the situation:

___

b) My positive affirmations for today are:

___

LOVE

I AM WORTHY OF LOVE,

I AM LOVING AND LOVABLE!

I AM STRONG ENOUGH TO GIVE LOVE,

I AM GRACIOUS TO RECEIVE LOVE!

LOVE

#61 Date:

Right now, I feel _____. I know/do not know (circle one) what triggered this feeling. My triggers as I know them are _____.

_____

_____

_____

_____

WHERE ARE MY THOUGHTS?

My thoughts are focused on my past/present/future (circle one), and they consist of _____.

_____

_____

_____

_____

To Feel Better I Will:

a) Choose the opposite behavior. (Use positive distractions list.)

b) Challenge my thoughts. (Just because I think a thought does not mean it's right!)

c) Limit access to triggers.

d) Silence my inner critic with positive self-talk.

e) Use coping skills. _____

_____

What Are My New Actions?

    a) New beliefs and thoughts about the situation:

    b) My positive affirmations for today are:

POSITIVE DISTRACTIONS LIST

1. Read a book.
2. Listen to music.
3. Go for a walk.
4. Call a friend.
5. Take a drive.
6. Exercise.
7. Meditate.
8. Watch a funny movie.
9. Do a crossword puzzle.
10. Decorate.
11. Plant a garden.
12. Play with your children.
13. Play with a pet.
14. Reorganize the room.
15. Clean out drawers.
16. Compliment someone.
17. Volunteer.
18. Encourage someone.
19. Visit a friend or family member.
20. Ride a bike.
21. Clean the house.
22. Hang out in nature.

23. Sit by the water (lake, pond, or beach).
24. Breathe deeply.
25. Hug yourself.
26. Draw.
27. Paint.
28. Play a video game.
29. Sing your favorite song.
30. Inhale your favorite candle or oil.
31. Take a warm bath with candles and music.
32. Dance.
33. Look at old photo albums.
34. Play an instrument.
35. Take a run.

MY FEELINGS LIST

1. **Happy**: cheerful, gratified, merry, gleeful, or lighthearted

2. **Sad**: out of sorts, despondent, depressed, gloomy, or dejected

3. **Angry**: irritated, resentful, annoyed, furious, or exasperated

4. **Fearful**: frightened, scared, afraid, panicky, or terrified

5. **Anxious**: worried, troubled, nervous, agitated, or uneasy

6. **Love**: passion, fondness, affectionate, adoration, or desire

7. **Calm**: quiet, peaceful, still, undisturbed, or restful

8. **Lonely**: isolated, alone, unloved, abandoned, or friendless

9. **Disgust**: detestation, aversion, revulsion, distaste, or disrelish

10. **Shame**: humiliation, embarrassment, indignity, or discomfort, mortification

11. **Guilt**: wrongdoing, misconduct, sin, blameworthiness, or criminality

12. **Embarrassed**: self-conscious, ashamed, blushing, disconcerted, or sheepish

13. **Apathy**: indifference, unconcerned, detachment, lack of interest, or passivity

14. **Envious**: covetous, desirous, jealous, spiteful, or bitter

15. **Shy**: timid, bashful, fearful, insecure, or withdrawn

16. **Surprised**: astonished, flabbergasted, amazed, shocked, or startled

17. **Depressed**: downcast, despondent, heavy-hearted, melancholy, or miserable

18. **Confused**: bewildered, disoriented, unbalanced, befuddled, or unhinged

19. **Bored**: weary, tired, restless, loss of interest, or impatient

20. **Frustrated**: annoyance, distress, anger, exasperation, or disappointment

- **My own feelings:**

___

___

___

___

___

___

www.ingramcontent.com/pod-product-compliance
Lightning Source LLC
Chambersburg PA
CBHW080848020526
44118CB00037B/2312